MIGRAINES DIET COOKBOOK

Delicious Recipes To Relieve Headache Pain, Reduce Triggers, And Improve Overall Wellness With Anti-Inflammatory And Nutrient-Rich Meals

DR ELIAN GRIFFIN

DISCLAIMER

The nutritional recommendations and recipes in this book are meant solely for informative reasons. They are not meant to replace the counsel, diagnosis, or care of a qualified medical expert. If you have any doubts about a medical condition or dietary requirements, you should always see your physician or another trained healthcare expert.

All reasonable efforts have been taken by the author and publisher to ensure that the information contained in this book is correct as of the date of publication. Recommendations may alter, though, as medical knowledge is always changing. When using any of the recipes or instructions found here, the user assumes all liability and assumes no risk, whether personal or otherwise. People who have certain dietary requirements or medical issues should speak with a healthcare provider for personalized guidance. The given recipes are only ideas; you may need to adjust them to suit your own nutritional needs, tastes, and tolerances.

When you use this book, you agree to release the publisher, the author, and their representatives from any liability for any claims, damages, liabilities, costs, or expenditures resulting from your use of the book.

TABLE OF CONTENTS

ABOUT THE BOOK

The "Migraines Diet Cookbook" is an invaluable tool for anyone attempting to navigate the challenges of controlling migraines with food choices. It starts by explaining the crucial role that diet plays in reducing migraine symptoms, stressing how particular foods can either precipitate or lessen episodes. By comprehending these subtleties, readers are empowered to create meals that complement their health objectives.

In addition to outlining the advantages of implementing a migraine-friendly diet, this cookbook offers helpful strategies for achieving success with its recipes. It presents readers with common ingredients that are crucial for managing migraines, guaranteeing clarity and simplicity in meal preparation.

With its extensive meal planning strategies and effective grocery shopping tips customized for migraine diets, the book gives readers the tools they need to simplify their cooking routines.

Essential to its efficacy, which explores the fundamentals of diets for migraineurs, providing an outline of typical triggers to stay away from and introducing foods that have therapeutic value? This basic information is supplemented with advice on meal planning strategies intended to maximize migraine relief; by incorporating these strategies, readers can proactively plan and cook meals that correspond with their dietary requirements and health goals.

The cookbook is made even more useful by the carefully selected recipes that cover a wide range of meal categories. From healthy breakfast options like protein-packed muffins and smoothie bowls to satisfying lunch ideas like salad combinations and flavorful grain bowls, every recipe is designed to balance nutrition and migraine relief. Dinner favorites include one-pot meals and veggie-packed options, so you can make satisfying choices that follow dietary guidelines.

The book provides a variety of between-meal snacks and appetizers that are low in calories and high in flavor. Energy bars made at home, nutrient-dense smoothies, and savory popcorn substitutes satisfy a wide range of palates while remaining true to migraine-safe guidelines. Desserts and treats are guilt-free treats that range from rich dark chocolate truffles to fruit-filled frozen yogurt bites, all made with ingredients selected to reduce migraine triggers.

Drink options are equally well-considered, with recipes for hydrating infused water, herbal tea blends that are well-known for relieving migraines, and invigorating coffee and tea types.

These choices guarantee that readers can stay hydrated and enjoy themselves without having to sacrifice their dietary objectives.

Acknowledging that social gatherings and eating out can be difficult, the cookbook offers menus for special occasions as well as useful advice on how to handle these situations safely. Lifestyle advice covers topics like stress reduction, how exercise can lessen the frequency of migraine attacks, and answering frequently asked questions with thorough FAQs and supplementary materials.

"Migraines Diet Cookbook" is a comprehensive manual that helps readers manage their condition through dietary decisions while also enabling them to enjoy a delicious and satisfying culinary experience that is in line with their health requirements. Whether making daily meal plans, preparing meals for special occasions, or looking for helpful lifestyle advice, this cookbook is a reliable travel companion for migraine relief and general well-being.

CHAPTER ONE

MIGRAINES DIET INTRODUCTION

KNOWING HOW DIET AFFECTS MIGRAINE MANAGEMENT

A critical component of migraine management is knowing how diet can affect the frequency and intensity of migraine attacks. For example, aged cheeses, processed meats, coffee, and alcohol are known triggers for many migraineurs, and these triggers can cause biochemical alterations in the brain that exacerbate migraine attacks.

On the other hand, a migraine-friendly diet aims to eliminate these triggers while highlighting foods high in magnesium, riboflavin (vitamin B2), and omega-3 fatty acids, which have been demonstrated to potentially lessen the frequency and severity of migraine attacks.

In addition, it is critical to keep blood sugar stable through regular meals and snacks because, for certain people, blood sugar fluctuations can cause migraines.

This dietary strategy tries to stabilize energy levels and prevent sharp drops in blood sugar, which are frequently linked to the onset of migraines. By knowing these concepts, people can start to modify their diet to effectively support migraine management.

Putting into practice a migraine-friendly diet entails not only avoiding triggers but also embracing foods that may prevent or alleviate symptoms. Examples of such foods include whole grains, lean proteins, healthy fats, and an abundance of fruits and vegetables. These foods offer vital nutrients without the added chemicals and preservatives that are frequently found in processed foods, which can aggravate migraine symptoms. By emphasizing nutrient-dense whole foods, people can promote overall health and possibly lessen the frequency and severity of migraines.

ADVANTAGES OF A DIET FRIENDLY TO MIGRAINES

Beyond just helping with symptoms, following a migraine-friendly diet has many advantages. A lot of the foods on these diets are high in antioxidants and anti-inflammatory compounds, which can help lower inflammation in the body as a whole. Chronic inflammation is thought to be involved in several illnesses, including migraines, so an anti-inflammatory diet is especially helpful.

A balanced diet for migraine sufferers can also help with overall energy levels and mood stability. People can avoid the energy crashes that come with processed and high-sugar foods, which helps people, maintain more stable energy throughout the day and can help reduce fatigue and migraine triggers. Better mental clarity and concentration can also be supported by this energy stability, which can be especially helpful during or after migraine attacks.

Following a migraine-friendly diet can also help improve digestive health because many of the foods are high in fiber and support gut health, which is becoming more and more important for overall health. A healthy gut can help the body absorb nutrients and support immune function, which can lessen overall stress on the body and lessen the chance of migraine triggers related to digestive disturbances.

HOW YOU CAN USE THIS COOKBOOK TO HELP

This cookbook provides a selection of recipes that are specifically created to avoid common migraine triggers while incorporating ingredients known to be beneficial for migraine sufferers. Each recipe is thoughtfully crafted to balance nutritional requirements with flavor and ease of preparation, making it accessible even for those who are new to cooking or managing dietary restrictions. The cookbook acts as a practical guide to implementing and maintaining a diet that supports migraine management.

In addition, the cookbook provides advice on how to make meal plans and prepare meals that will make switching to a migraine-friendly diet easier. It also offers advice on how to stock a pantry that is migraine-friendly, choose fresh ingredients, and modify recipes to suit specific dietary requirements and preferences.

Finally, by giving detailed instructions and nutritional data for every recipe, the cookbook gives people the power to take charge of their diet and how it affects their migraine symptoms.

In addition, the cookbook promotes experimentation and adaptation, acknowledging that dietary preferences and sensitivities can differ greatly among migraineurs. It invites readers to investigate novel flavors and ingredients while adhering to the fundamentals of a diet that is migraine-friendly. In the end, this tool seeks to assist people on their path to improved migraine management by providing them with satisfying and satisfying meals.

ADVICE FOR USING THE RECIPES SUCCESSFULLY

Planning meals ensures that ingredients are on hand and meals can be prepared without stress or last-minute decisions, which not only saves time but also lessens the temptation to reach for convenience foods that may trigger migraines.

Practical strategies and tips are essential to successfully implementing a migraine-friendly diet and maintaining consistency.

Adding new recipes and ingredients to your diet gradually will also help you see how they affect your migraine patterns. You can also fine-tune your dietary choices over time by keeping a food diary, which can help you identify potential triggers or patterns in your migraine occurrences. Finally, following your body's signals and customizing recipes to your unique tastes and tolerances will help you feel more satisfied and stick to your diet.

In addition, mixing things up can help you avoid getting bored with your food and guarantee that you are getting enough nutrients. You can also maximize the benefits of a migraine-friendly diet and improve your overall health by experimenting in the kitchen with different cooking techniques, herbs, and spices to give your food more depth and flavor without using additives that trigger migraines.

The use of particular foods that are known to support migraine management and reduce triggers is emphasized in migraine diets. These foods include fresh fruits and vegetables, which are high in antioxidants, vitamins, and minerals that support overall health and reduce inflammation; citrus fruits, leafy greens, and berries are especially helpful because of their high vitamin C and other bioactive compound content.

Furthermore, whole grains like quinoa, brown rice, and oats are high in fiber, which promotes digestive health and lowers the risk of gastrointestinal disturbances that in certain people can cause migraines. These grains also contain complex carbohydrates that help stabilize blood sugar levels and prevent energy crashes.

Because they are lower in risk of causing migraine attacks than processed meats, lean proteins—fish, poultry, and tofu, for example—are mainstays of migraine diets because they offer essential amino acids for muscle repair and general health without the added chemicals and preservatives that are frequently present in processed protein sources.

Another essential component of diets for migraine prevention is healthy fats, like those found in avocados, nuts, seeds, and olive oil. These fats offer omega-3 fatty acids and monounsaturated fats, which support brain health and have anti-inflammatory qualities. Including these fats in meals can help balance cholesterol levels and improve cardiovascular health, both of which are critical for overall well-being and migraine prevention.

Finally, because of their anti-inflammatory and antioxidant qualities, herbs and spices like garlic, ginger, and turmeric are commonly used in migraine-friendly cooking. These ingredients not only enhance the flavor and complexity of meals but also add to the overall health benefits of a well-balanced diet that minimizes migraine triggers.

CHAPTER TWO

UNDERSTANDING MIGRAINE DIETS

AN OVERVIEW OF FOODS TO AVOID AND TRIGGERS FOR MIGRAINE

A person's diet is a critical component in controlling the triggers of their migraines. Aged cheeses, processed meats, and foods containing monosodium glutamate (MSG) are common foods that cause migraines because they contain high levels of tyramine or other additives that can cause migraine symptoms. Alcohol, particularly red wine and beer, can also be a major cause of migraines because of their high histamine content.

Keeping a detailed food diary can help identify and eliminate personal triggers from your diet. Certain ingredients in everyday foods, such as coffee, tea, and chocolate, can trigger migraines. While small amounts of caffeine can help alleviate headaches for some people, excessive consumption can cause withdrawal headaches. Artificial sweeteners like aspartame and foods with high nitrate content, like hot dogs and deli meats, should also be avoided.

Reducing processed foods (fast food included) is recommended because they frequently have unidentified additives and preservatives that can cause migraines; choosing fresh, whole foods and cooking at home gives you more control over what you put in your food and lowers the chance that you'll unintentionally consume a trigger; staying hydrated and adhering to regular eating schedules also help prevent migraine episodes.

OVERVIEW OF FOODS THAT ARE MIGRAINE-FRIENDLY

Fresh, natural, and minimally processed foods are the cornerstones of a migraine-friendly diet, which also emphasizes whole grains, lean proteins, and fresh fruits and vegetables. Foods high in magnesium, like spinach, quinoa, and pumpkin seeds, are especially helpful because magnesium has been shown to lessen the frequency and intensity of migraines.

Omega-3 fatty acids, which are found in fish like salmon and mackerel, can also help reduce inflammation and support brain health.

Including a range of vibrant fruits and vegetables guarantees a sufficient intake of the vitamins and minerals required for general well-being and the prevention of migraines.

Vegetables such as sweet potatoes, carrots, and leafy greens are great options. Lean meats like turkey, chicken, lentils, and chickpeas are great sources of protein and offer essential nutrients without the added chemicals and preservatives found in processed foods.

In addition, drinking lots of water throughout the day can help prevent dehydration, which is a common migraine trigger. Herbal teas, particularly those with calming properties like peppermint or chamomile, can also be beneficial. By emphasizing these nourishing, whole foods, people can create a balanced diet that supports migraine management.

Preparing meals ahead of time helps people avoid making impulsive food choices that could contain trigger ingredients. It also makes it easier to include a range of migraine-friendly foods, resulting in a balanced diet that promotes overall health. Eating a healthy, migraine-free diet is made possible by meal planning.

Making a weekly meal plan can make grocery shopping easier and less stressful than preparing meals every day. Knowing exactly what to eat when helps people stick to a regular eating schedule, which is important for blood sugar regulation and avoiding migraines brought on by hunger. Meal prep, or cooking large quantities of food ahead of time and storing it for later, is a great way to save time and guarantee that there are always healthy options available.

Additionally, meal planning makes it easier to control portion sizes and nutritional content. It guarantees that every meal is balanced, including the required amounts of fats, proteins, and carbohydrates in addition to vital vitamins and minerals. This methodical approach not only helps prevent migraine triggers but also encourages a healthier lifestyle by making it simpler to follow dietary guidelines and lessen the frequency and severity of migraine attacks.

The key to using this cookbook for a migraine diet effectively is learning how to incorporate the recipes into your daily routine while avoiding common triggers. To begin, become acquainted with the various sections of the cookbook.

Each section is meant to provide a range of meal options, such as breakfast, lunch, dinner, and snacks. All of the recipes are made to be nutrient-dense and free of common migraine triggers, so meal planning will be made easier.

This cookbook includes substitution suggestions to help you tailor meals to your specific dietary needs.

Preparing a few recipes ahead of time and storing them can ensure you always have migraine-friendly meals ready to go, reducing the temptation to turn to potentially triggering convenience foods. When trying new recipes, pay attention to portion sizes and ingredient lists. If you are sensitive to certain foods, even those considered generally safe for migraines, modify the recipes accordingly.

If you follow these guidelines, you can effectively manage your diet and lower your risk of migraines while enjoying a diverse and delicious range of meals. You can also use the cookbook as a guide when creating your weekly meal plan. By choosing a variety of recipes, you can ensure a balanced diet that covers all necessary nutrients. The cookbook also offers tips on ingredient sourcing and preparation techniques to maximize nutritional benefits.

TIPS FOR GROCERY PURCHASING FOR MIGRAINE DIETS

When grocery shopping for a migraine diet, choose whole, fresh foods and steer clear of anything that might trigger a migraine. Make a detailed shopping list based on your weekly meal plan to help you stay focused and steer clear of impulsive purchases that might contain harmful additives. When possible, choose organic produce to minimize your exposure to pesticides that may trigger migraines.

For protein sources, choose fresh, unprocessed options like turkey, chicken, fish, and plant-based proteins like beans and lentils. Steer clear of processed meats and those with nitrates or nitrites.

Choose plain, unsweetened dairy products in the dairy aisle, and if you have sensitivity to cow's milk, consider alternatives like almond or oat milk. Always read labels to identify hidden ingredients that may cause migraines.

A good portion of your cart should be made up of fruits and vegetables. Look for a wide range of colors and varieties to ensure a wide range of nutrients. If certain fruits, like bananas or avocados, are known triggers for you, proceed with caution when buying them. Stock up on whole grains, like quinoa, brown rice, and oats, and steer clear of packaged snacks and refined grains. Being aware of your surroundings and alert when shopping will help ensure that your kitchen is stocked with migraine-friendly foods, making it easier to follow your eating plan.

CHAPTER THREE

MEAL PREPARATION AND PLANNING

STRATEGIES FOR WEEKLY MEAL PLANNING

A calendar or meal planning app can be used to map out your week, ensuring a balance of nutrients and migraine-safe foods. Aim to include a variety of fruits, vegetables, lean proteins, and whole grains, and avoid known migraine triggers like processed foods, artificial sweeteners, and aged cheeses.

Knowing your dietary needs and preferences is the first step in creating an effective weekly meal plan, especially when managing migraines.

Meal planning should be flexible to allow for unforeseen changes in your schedule. Recipes that feature common ingredients should be chosen to reduce waste and streamline preparation. For example, if you plan to use chicken for a stir-fry on Monday, you may use it for a salad or wrap later in the week. You should also mix quick meals with meals that can be prepared ahead of time, such as casseroles or soups, so that you have healthy options even on your busiest days.

Meal planning can be more effective if you make a master list of your favorite migraine-safe recipes and rotate them regularly. This will help you plan more efficiently and guarantee that you have a variety of meals throughout the month. You should also always pay attention to portion control and balance, and you can modify your plan in response to new triggers or dietary requirements that may arise.

TIPS FOR BATCH COOKING ON BUSY DAYS

Preparing and cooking meals in bulk, then portioning them into individual servings using easily stored clear containers or bags labeled with the contents and date will help you make sure you always have nutritious, migraine-friendly meals on hand, even on your busiest days. Start by choosing a few adaptable recipes that can be easily scaled up, like soups, stews, and casseroles. Set aside a specific day of the week, like Sunday, for your batch cooking session.

Aim for multi-cooking to save time and energy. For example, roast a large batch of vegetables while a stew simmers on the stovetop. To maximize efficiency during your batch cooking session, prep all your ingredients ahead of time.

This includes chopping vegetables, marinating proteins, and measuring out spices. Utilize kitchen appliances like rice cookers, slow cookers, or instant pots to free up time and space.

After cooking and portioning, keep your meals in the freezer or refrigerator for convenient access during the week. Invest in high-quality, airtight containers to maintain freshness and prevent freezer burn. Rotate your meals, eating the oldest ones first to prevent spoilage.

Batch cooking not only saves time but also guarantees that you always have wholesome, migraine-safe options on hand, which lessens the temptation to reach for processed, unhealthy convenience foods.

Making an effective grocery shopping list is essential to sticking to a migraine-safe diet and saving time and money. Begin by structuring your list according to your weekly meal plan, dividing it into sections like produce, proteins, grains, and dairy. This way, you make sure you only buy what you need, cutting down on wasteful spending and food waste. Before you shop, make sure to check your pantry and refrigerator to make sure you don't buy duplicates.

Prioritize whole, fresh foods over processed ones that can aggravate migraines. Stock up on a range of fruits and vegetables, lean proteins (like fish or chicken), and whole grains (like brown rice or quinoa). For energy boosts during the day, choose migraine-friendly snacks (like almonds, seeds, and fresh fruit). Buy staples (like rice, oats, and beans) in bulk to cut costs and packaging waste.

You can make grocery shopping a quick and efficient part of your meal planning routine by organizing your shopping list based on how your favorite grocery store is laid out; grouping similar items to minimize backtracking and save time; shopping during off-peak hours to avoid crowds and reduce stress; and taking advantage of grocery delivery or pickup services to ensure you get everything you need.

The quality and safety of your migraine-friendly meals depend on how well you store and freeze them. To start, buy some good, airtight, freezer-safe, label-friendly containers. Then, portion your meals according to your needs, whether you're serving a family or just yourself. This will keep the meals fresh and make it easy to thaw and reheat individual portions as needed.

Aim to use frozen meals within three months for best quality, although many can last longer if stored properly. Label each container with the date and contents to keep track of what you have and when it was prepared. Make sure meals have cooled completely before placing them in the freezer.

This avoids condensation and ice crystals, which can lead to freezer burn and compromise the taste and texture of your food.

In the fridge, most cooked meals will be kept for up to four days. To prolong their shelf life, consider vacuum sealing, which removes air and prevents spoilage.

By following these storage and freezing guidelines, you can make sure that your migraine-friendly meals stay delicious and safe to eat, even when prepared in advance. To store leftovers, use the same principles of portioning and labeling. Store leftovers in airtight containers and place them in the coldest part of your fridge, usually the back.

HOW TO MODIFY RECIPES TO FIT YOUR TASTE

When it comes to managing migraines, it's important to modify recipes to suit your tastes and dietary requirements. To start, identify common migraine triggers in recipes, like aged cheeses, processed meats, and artificial additives.

Replace these with migraine-safe substitutions, like fresh herbs, lean proteins, and natural flavorings. For instance, you can use fresh lemon juice instead of vinegar or substitute younger, milder cheese for aged cheese.

When modifying recipes, take your dietary needs and taste preferences into account. If you have gluten sensitivity or prefer a particular kind of protein, look for appropriate gluten-free alternatives. For example, you can replace pasta with quinoa or rice, or use tofu or beans as a source of protein in vegetarian dishes.

You can also try different herbs and spices to add flavor without using potentially triggering ingredients. You can also keep a record of successful substitutions to make meal planning and cooking easier in the future.

Maintaining the harmony of flavors and textures is crucial when adjusting recipes. Cooking times and techniques should also be adjusted to get the desired results. For instance, if tofu is being used in place of chicken, marinate it longer to improve flavor absorption. Don't be afraid to get creative and customize the recipe; with practice, you'll become more adept at adjusting recipes to fit your migraine-safe diet, guaranteeing that you enjoy satisfying and tasty meals that meet your health requirements.

INVIGORATING BOWLS OF SMOOTHIES

Smoothie bowls are a great way to start the day off right with a healthy dose of nutrients. To make a simple smoothie bowl, blend a combination of frozen fruits (bananas, berries, and mangoes) with a small amount of your favorite liquid (almond milk, coconut water, etc.) until the smoothie is thick and creamy. Transfer the smoothie to a bowl and use a spoon to smooth the top.

Next, add a variety of toppings to your smoothie bowl to add both texture and extra nutrients. Some popular toppings are sliced fresh fruit for extra vitamins, chia seeds for a dose of omega-3 fatty acids, and granola for crunch. You can also try experimenting with different combinations to find your favorite combination of flavors and textures.

Lastly, to add even more energy and benefits to your smoothie bowl for migraine sufferers, think about adding anti-inflammatory ingredients.

Top your smoothie bowl with dark leafy greens like kale or spinach, or add a teaspoon of turmeric or ginger to the smoothie base. These additions can help reduce inflammation and give you a sustained energy boost, so you can start your day off right.

QUICK AND HEALTHFUL OATMEAL TYPES

A healthy and adaptable breakfast choice, oatmeal can be made quickly to your tastes. To make oatmeal, start with rolled oats, which you can cook with water or milk on the stovetop or in the microwave until the consistency you want; if you want a creamier texture, use half water and half milk.

Add a variety of mix-ins to your oatmeal to increase its nutritional value. Dried or fresh fruits like raisins, apples, and walnuts add vitamins and natural sweetness.

Nuts and seeds like almonds, walnuts, and flaxseeds offer healthy fats and protein. A spoonful of Greek yogurt can add extra protein and creaminess.

You can naturally sweeten your oatmeal with a drizzle of maple syrup or honey. You can also add spices like nutmeg or cinnamon to enhance its flavor.

If you want your oatmeal to be migraine-friendly, think about including ingredients that are known to help with migraines. For example, ground flaxseed or chia seeds, which are high in omega-3 fatty acids and have anti-inflammatory properties, can be a tasty addition that also contains magnesium, which may help reduce migraine symptoms. Making your oatmeal the night before as overnight oats is another great way to save time and make sure you have a healthy breakfast ready to go in the morning.

HIGH-PROTEIN MORNING MUFFINS

For busy mornings, these high-protein muffins are a quick and healthy option. Preheat the oven to 350°F (175°C), line a muffin tin with paper liners or grease it with cooking spray, and whisk together whole wheat flour, baking powder, and a pinch of salt in a large bowl.

Beat the eggs, Greek yogurt, and your preferred sweetener (such as honey or maple syrup) in a separate bowl.

Mix the wet and dry ingredients; fold in protein-rich ingredients such as chopped nuts, seeds, and a small handful of shredded cheese; you can also mix in grated veggies (like carrots or zucchini) or diced cooked meats (like bacon or ham) for extra nutrition and flavor; spoon batter into prepared muffin tin, filling each cup about two-thirds full.

To ensure that you have a well-balanced and high-protein start to your day, bake the muffins for 20 to 25 minutes, or until a toothpick inserted into the center comes out clean.

Let them cool slightly before removing them from the tin. These muffins can be frozen for longer-term storage or kept in an airtight container for several days.

A refreshing and nutritious way to start the day, fresh fruit parfaits is an easy breakfast that looks good. To make them, first choose a variety of fresh fruits, like berries, kiwi, mango, and banana. Next, wash and slice the fruits into bite-sized pieces, and set them aside in separate bowls.

To assemble the parfait, place a spoonful of yogurt (I recommend Greek yogurt because it's thick and creamy and high in protein) in the bottom of a glass or bowl, then top with a layer of your preferred fruits and a scattering of granola for crunch.

Continue layering the yogurt and fruit until the container is full, then top with a dollop of yogurt and a final scattering of fruit and granola.

These parfaits are delicious and nutritious breakfast options that can be prepared ahead of time and refrigerated. For extra flavor and health benefits, try drizzling a little honey or a sprinkling of seeds like chia or flax between the layers. Fresh mint leaves or a dash of cinnamon can also enhance the flavor profile.

ENERGIZING WRAPS FOR BREAKFAST

A healthy and filling way to eat on the go is with energizing breakfast wraps. First, preheat a whole wheat tortilla or wrap it in a dry skillet over medium heat until it becomes pliable. In the meantime, make your filling by scrambling eggs with diced bell peppers, onions, and spinach in a nonstick skillet until the vegetables are soft and the eggs are cooked through.

Place a generous spoonful of the egg and vegetable mixture in the center of the warmed tortilla; top with a dollop of Greek yogurt, cooked bacon or sausage, or shredded cheese for extra flavor and protein. Roll the tortilla tightly, folding in the sides as you go, to form a tidy, handheld wrap.

Breakfast wraps can be made ahead of time, wrapped in foil or parchment paper, and stored in the refrigerator for a quick, grab-and-go option that guarantees you start your day with a nutritious, energizing meal. For a migraine-friendly twist, consider adding anti-inflammatory ingredients like avocado slices, which provide healthy fats, or a sprinkle of turmeric or cumin for added flavor and health benefits.

EASY SALAD COMBINATIONS TO ALLEVIATE MIGRAINES

Choosing ingredients with anti-inflammatory and anti-migraine qualities is key when making simple salad combinations for migraine relief. Begin with a base of leafy greens, such as spinach or kale, which are high in magnesium and can help lessen the frequency of migraines.

Add colorful vegetables, like bell peppers, carrots, and cucumbers, to your salad to boost its vitamin and antioxidant content. Finally, add proteins, like grilled chicken, chickpeas, or hard-boiled eggs, to make sure your salad is substantial and well-balanced.

Nuts like almonds or walnuts not only add a satisfying crunch but also serve as a good source of magnesium and healthy fats, which are essential in a migraine-friendly diet. Berries like blueberries or strawberries can provide a natural sweetness and additional antioxidants.

Avocado, olive oil, and seeds are healthy fats that support brain health and reduce inflammation, and can improve the migraine-relieving properties of the salad.

Sprinkle some fresh herbs, such as parsley or cilantro, over your salad to help with digestion and to add flavor without the heavy dressings; alternatively, make your dressing with olive oil, lemon juice, and a little honey or mustard for a homemade, healthful option. With careful ingredient selection, you can make tasty, satisfying, migraine-friendly salads.

HEALTHY RECIPES FOR GRAIN BOWLS

A flavorful broth adds taste and nutrients to your cooked grains, which you then fluff with a fork and let cool slightly before assembling your bowl. Quinoa, brown rice, and farro are excellent base grains that arc high in fiber and provide sustained energy without aggravating migraines. Nourishing grain bowls are a flexible and satisfying option for a migraine-friendly lunch.

Add a protein source, such as grilled tofu, chickpeas, or shredded chicken, to make the bowl more filling and well-balanced. On top of your grain base, add a variety of vegetables, both raw and cooked, to ensure a mix of textures and flavors. Roasted sweet potatoes, steamed broccoli, sautéed spinach, and fresh cherry tomatoes are excellent choices that offer vitamins, minerals, and antioxidants.

Add a few fresh herbs, a sprinkling of seeds, and a drizzle of a migraine-friendly dressing (try a creamy avocado-lime dressing or a basic tahini dressing made with tahini, lemon juice, water, and a pinch of salt). These garnishes not only add flavor to your grain bowl but also boost its nutritional content, keeping you full and migraine-free.

DELICIOUS SOUP RECIPES

Cooking with fresh, health-promoting ingredients is a great way to create flavorful soups that fit into a migraine-friendly diet. Start with a base of low-sodium vegetable or chicken broth, which gives the soup a nice base without adding too much salt, which can aggravate migraines. Then, add aromatic vegetables like celery, onions, and garlic, sautéed in olive oil to release their natural flavors and form the soup's base.

Add color, nutrients, and texture to the soup by adding a variety of vegetables like carrots, zucchini, and leafy greens like spinach or kale. If you'd like to make the soup more substantial, add beans, lentils, or small pasta shapes that cook quickly and absorb the flavors of the broth. Season the soup with anti-inflammatory herbs and spices like turmeric, ginger, and parsley, which can help relieve migraine symptoms.

Simmer until everything is soft and the flavors have blended. If you want a creamy texture without dairy, you can blend some of the soup and then add it back in, or you can add coconut milk for a rich, migraine-friendly option. Serve the soup hot, garnished with fresh herbs and lemon juice to savor the flavors and add even more nutrition.

A migraine-friendly lunch requires careful ingredient selection to avoid common migraine triggers. Lean proteins like grilled chicken or turkey, or plant-based options like hummus or black bean spread, are preferable to processed meats and cheeses, which can contain preservatives and additives that may trigger migraines. Whole-grain bread or wraps are a good place to start because they provide fiber and essential nutrients.

Add a variety of fresh vegetables—leafy greens, tomatoes, cucumbers, and bell peppers are great options—to your sandwich or wrap to add crunch, flavor, and nutrients. Avocado slices or a smear of guacamole, which provides healthy fats that support brain health, add even more flavor and consider adding sprouts or microgreens for a nutrient-dense topping that enhances the overall flavor profile.

Use migraine-friendly homemade spreads and condiments to keep your sandwich or wrap tasty and visually appealing. A light vinaigrette, tahini spread, or yogurt-based dressing can provide flavor and moisture without the need for store-bought items. Tightly wrap or use a toothpick to hold your sandwich together. These choices will guarantee that you have a satisfying, migraine-safe lunch that is well-balanced and nutritious.

Producing inventive salad dressings and vinaigrettes at home gives you the advantage of being in charge of the ingredients and avoiding possible migraine triggers present in store-bought options. To begin, use a basic vinaigrette formula: three parts oil to one part acid. For its anti-inflammatory qualities, use extra virgin olive oil, and combine it with balsamic vinegar, apple cider vinegar, or lemon juice, each of which has distinct flavors and health benefits.

Add more flavorings and ingredients to your vinaigrette: fresh herbs such as basil, dill, and cilantro can give your dressing brightness and depth; a small amount of honey or maple syrup can add sweetness and balance the acidity while adding complexity to the flavor profile; and yogurt or mustard can add tanginess and a creamy texture without dairy or mayonnaise.

Try experimenting with different oils and vinegar for more daring dressings; walnut, sesame, or flaxseed oils can impart distinct flavors and offer additional health benefits; these can be combined with citrus juices, such as orange or lime, to create novel and refreshing vinaigrettes; whisk all ingredients until thoroughly combined, or shake in a jar for ease of use; with homemade dressings, you can enjoy flavorful, fresh, migraine-friendly salads that are customized to your preferences.

HEALTHY ONE-POT DINNERS

One-pot meals are a lifesaver for hectic evenings because they are quick and easy to prepare without compromising on taste or nutrition. To begin, choose an ingredient that will serve as the base of your dish, like rice, quinoa, or pasta. In a large pot, sauté onions and garlic in olive oil until fragrant, then add your base of choice along with a variety of chopped vegetables, like bell peppers, carrots, and zucchini. Add enough broth to cover the ingredients and simmer until the base is tender and the flavors have blended.

Lean meats such as turkey or chicken can be added to the pot after they have been browned in a separate pan. Alternatively, beans or lentils can be added as a vegetarian source of protein that complements the other ingredients. Season with herbs and spices like thyme, rosemary, and a small amount of salt and pepper to taste. Stir occasionally to keep the dish from sticking and cook until everything is soft and well-combined.

Finally, stir in a handful of fresh spinach or kale and let it wilt from the residual heat to add a nutritious green element to your meal. Serve your one-pot meal straight from the pot for a minimally messy, satisfying, and healthful dinner that's ideal for migraine sufferers trying to control their migraines with food.

The definition of comfort food, casseroles is a delicious way to combine different ingredients into a cohesive, baked dish. To make a casserole, start with some prepared base, like cooked quinoa, brown rice, or whole-grain pasta, and spread it evenly in a greased baking dish. Then, top with cooked vegetables, like sautéed broccoli, mushrooms, and bell peppers.

Lean ground turkey or shredded chicken that has been well-seasoned and cooked through can be used as the protein. If you're a vegetarian, you can also use black beans or tofu. After layering the protein over the vegetables, make a creamy sauce with low-sodium chicken broth, almond milk, and a small bit of cornstarch for thickening. Finally, pour the sauce evenly over the layers of the casserole to make sure every bite is moist and flavorful.

This dish is great for making ahead and reheating, providing a cozy and migraine-friendly dinner option. Top the casserole with a light sprinkle of cheese, such as shredded mozzarella or a dairy-free alternative, and bake in a preheated oven at 350°F (175°C) for about 30-40 minutes, or until the top is golden and bubbling. Let it cool slightly before serving to allow the flavors to meld and the casserole to set.

SIMPLE STIR-FRY DISHES

Recipes for stir-fries are easy to make and adapt, making them ideal for preparing a migraine-friendly dinner. To begin, prepare your ingredients by slicing a variety of colorful veggies into bite-sized pieces, such as bell peppers, broccoli, snap peas, and carrots. You can also thinly slice your protein of choice, such as tofu, beef strips, or chicken breast.

Lightly oil a large skillet or wok over medium-high heat; once hot, add your protein and cook until browned and cooked through, then take it out of the pan and set aside. In the same pan, add a little more oil if necessary and add your vegetables; stir-fry for a few minutes, just until they are tender-crisp, but still have some bite and color, and add the minced garlic and ginger for flavor, stirring all the time to avoid burning.

Put the cooked protein back in the pan and add a simple sauce consisting of low-sodium soy sauce, a little honey, and a squeeze of fresh lemon juice. Toss to coat evenly and cook for an additional minute to let the flavors meld. Serve your stir-fry over brown rice or quinoa for a complete, healthy, and quick-to-make dinner that's perfect for weeknights.

TYPES OF BAKED FISH AND CHICKEN

Preheat your oven to 375°F (190°C). Line a baking sheet with parchment paper to prevent sticking and make cleanup easier. Start with fresh, high-quality fish fillets like salmon, cod, tilapia, or chicken breasts and thighs. Baked fish and chicken dishes are great options for those following a migraine-friendly diet, providing lean protein without excessive fat.

When baking fish, spread some olive oil over the fillets on the prepared baking sheet, season with salt, pepper, and herbs like dill, parsley, or thyme, and top with lemon slices for a zesty pop of flavor. Bake for 12 to 15 minutes, depending on the thickness of the fillets, or until the fish is opaque and flakes easily with a fork.

To make a balanced, headache-friendly meal that is both satisfying and simple to prepare, season the chicken breasts or thighs with olive oil, salt, pepper, and your preferred spices such as paprika, garlic powder, or rosemary.

Arrange them on the baking sheet and bake for 25 to 30 minutes, or until the internal temperature of the chicken reaches 165°F (74°C) and the juices run clear.

Including more veggies in your dinner can greatly help a migraine-friendly diet by providing necessary nutrients without having ingredients that trigger migraines. Start with a variety of fresh vegetables, like bell peppers, zucchini, sweet potatoes, and leafy greens like spinach and kale. Toss the vegetables in olive oil, salt, and pepper, and roast them in the oven at 400°F (200°C) for 20 to 25 minutes, or until they are soft and starting to caramelize.

A hearty vegetable stew is another veggie-packed option. First, sauté onions, garlic, and celery in a large pot until softened. Next, add chopped vegetables, like carrots, potatoes, and tomatoes, along with vegetable broth.

Season with a pinch of salt and pepper and herbs like thyme and bay leaves. Simmer the stew for 30 to 40 minutes, or until the vegetables are tender and the flavors have developed. If you want to add extra protein, you may want to add beans or lentils.

Think about preparing pasta dishes with vegetables, such as spaghetti squash or zucchini noodles. Combine the cooked noodles with a homemade tomato sauce made with fresh tomatoes, garlic, and basil. Serve with sautéed mushrooms, spinach, and a sprinkle of Parmesan cheese or another dairy-free cheese substitute. These nutritious dinners are not only satisfying but also promote a diet that is good for migraine sufferers.

MAKE YOUR ENERGY BARS AND BITS

It's easy and satisfying to make your energy bars and bites, especially if you suffer from migraines. To begin, gather migraine-friendly ingredients like rolled oats, almond butter, honey, and dried fruits. In a big bowl, thoroughly combine two cups of rolled oats, half a cup of almond butter, and a third of a cup of honey. Add a cup of chopped dried fruits, such as dates or apricots, for flavor and texture. Just make sure the dried fruits are free of sulfites, which can aggravate migraines.

After mixing everything thoroughly, press the mixture firmly into a lined baking dish, making sure the thickness is even. Refrigerate the dish for at least an hour so the bars can solidify. Once chilled, cut the mixture into bite-sized bars or squares. These can be kept in the refrigerator for up to a week in an airtight container, providing a quick and easy snack option that helps maintain steady energy levels without causing migraines.

Try experimenting with different flavors and add-ins to keep your snacks interesting and in line with your dietary preferences. These homemade energy bars are great for on-the-go snacks because they provide a balanced combination of protein, healthy fats, and carbohydrates that help prevent migraine symptoms. For example, you can add a handful of unsweetened shredded coconut or a tablespoon of cocoa powder for a chocolatey touch.

PLATES OF FRESH VEGETABLES WITH DIP

A healthy snack that is also migraine-friendly is a fresh veggie and dip platter. To start, gather a variety of vibrant, fresh vegetables, such as carrots, celery, cucumber, cherry tomatoes, and bell peppers. Wash and chop the vegetables into bite-sized pieces for easy presentation and dipping. If at all possible, choose organic produce to avoid pesticide residues, which can occasionally trigger migraines.

A classic hummus made with chickpeas, tahini, lemon juice, garlic, and olive oil is a great option for the dips;

another delicious and migraine-friendly option is a Greek yogurt dip made with fresh herbs like parsley and dill, lemon juice, and a pinch of salt. These dips not only enhance the flavor of the vegetables but also provide extra nutrients like protein and healthy fats.

Arrange the veggies and dips in a visually appealing manner, arranging colors that go well together to create a visually appealing display. This platter can be made in advance and refrigerated until ready to serve, which makes it a convenient option for entertaining as well as casual snacking. The crunchy veggies and creamy dips make for a satisfying snack that is low in calories and high in nutrients, all without the risk of aggravating migraines.

RICH IN NUTRIENT SMOOTHIES

For those on a migraine-friendly diet, nutrient-dense smoothies are a quick and flexible solution. Begin with a base of migraine-safe liquids, like water, almond milk, or coconut water. To this base, add a variety of fresh or frozen fruits, making sure they are low in tyramine, a common migraine trigger. Spinach, bananas, and blueberries are great options because they offer a range of vitamins and minerals without aggravating migraine symptoms.

Add protein and healthy fats to make the smoothie more balanced and filling. You can add the necessary protein with a tablespoon of almond butter or a scoop of plain Greek yogurt, and the healthy fats with a small avocado or a handful of chia seeds. Blend these ingredients until smooth, adding more liquid if needed to adjust the thickness.

If you want to add even more nutrients, you can add a teaspoon of ground flaxseeds or a handful of baby spinach, which are high in magnesium and omega-3 fatty acids, respectively.

Try blending different combinations of flavors to make your smoothies interesting and fun. For example, try blending pineapple, coconut milk, and a small amount of fresh ginger for a tropical twist, or try blending strawberries, blueberries, almond milk, and a dash of vanilla extract for a creamy berry blend. These smoothies are easy to make and a great way to maintain a migraine-safe diet while providing you with sustained energy throughout the day.

TASTY POPCORN SAFE FOR MIGRAINES

A tasty and simple snack that satisfies your cravings and dietary requirements, making savory migraine-safe popcorn starts with organic kernels because conventional kernels may contain pesticides and other additives. Heat a tablespoon of coconut oil or olive oil in a large pot over medium heat, then add a half-cup of popcorn kernels and cover the pot with a lid, shaking it occasionally to avoid burning. Heat until the popping slows down, then remove from heat.

Instead of artificial flavors, use natural herbs and spices to create a cheesy flavor without the dairy that triggers migraines in some people. Alternatively, combine dried herbs like oregano, thyme, and rosemary with a little garlic powder to create a savory herbal blend.

Toss the freshly popped popcorn with your preferred seasoning while it's still warm to ensure an even coating.

As a versatile snack that's simple to make and can be seasoned to your taste, popcorn is best enjoyed fresh, though it can be kept in an airtight container for a few days if necessary. This homemade version of popcorn is free of artificial ingredients and preservatives that are often found in store-bought popcorn, making it a safer option for those who are prone to migraines while still providing a satisfying, crunchy snack.

EASY PICKLES AND DIPS

A quick and easy way to enjoy migraine-friendly snacks is to make quick pickles and dips. For the pickles, use migraine-resistant vegetables like cucumbers, carrots, and radishes; thinly slice the vegetables and put them in a glass jar. In a small saucepan, heat one cup of water, one cup of white vinegar, and a tablespoon of salt until the salt dissolves. Pour this brine over the vegetables in the jar, making sure they are completely submerged.

Allow the pickles to sit at room temperature for one hour before refrigerating them. Enjoy within hours, or even days.

Just use good, whole-food ingredients for the dips: ripe avocados, lime juice, salt, and minced garlic for classic guacamole; cannellini beans blended with olive oil, lemon juice, and cumin for a simple white bean dip; both are very easy to make and go well with a variety of fresh veggies and wholehearted crackers.

Making your pickles and dips will ensure that they are free of artificial additives and preservatives, keeping your diet wholesome and migraine-safe. These easy recipes are great to prepare ahead of time and keep in the refrigerator for any time you want a healthy snack. They offer a satisfying balance of creamy textures and tangy, fresh flavors.

RICH DARK CHOCOLATE CANDIES

Because it is less likely to cause headaches than milk chocolate, dark chocolate is a wonderful indulgence for migraine sufferers. To make an easy yet incredibly rich dark chocolate treat, melt some high-quality dark chocolate (at least 70% cocoa) over a double boiler until it is smooth. Then, pour the melted chocolate into silicone molds and, while it is still warm, sprinkle in some chopped nuts, seeds, or dried fruits of your choice. Then, let the chocolate cool and harden in the refrigerator for about half an hour. After they are set, remove the molds and savor these rich, bite-sized treats.

Dark chocolate avocado truffles are a unique take on the traditional chocolate truffle. First, puree ripe avocados; then, add melted dark chocolate and a small dash of vanilla extract. After well combined, set the mixture in the fridge for an hour. Next, scoop the mixture into small balls with a small scoop and roll them in cocoa powder, finely chopped nuts, or shredded coconut. These truffles are rich, creamy, and full of healthy fats that are beneficial to both the body and the mind.

Dark chocolate bark is a delightful way to enjoy dark chocolate. Simply spread melted dark chocolate thinly on a baking sheet lined with parchment paper, and then sprinkle with a variety of toppings (like sea salt, crushed peppermint candies, or freeze-dried berries) before it sets. Then, put the baking sheet in the refrigerator to harden, and once it's firm, break the bark into irregular pieces. This simple treat is visually appealing and offers a delightful mix of flavors and textures with every bite.

BITS OF FROZEN YOGURT WITH FRUIT INFUSION

For those who manage migraines, fruit-infused frozen yogurt bites are a refreshing and healthy dessert option. To make them, first choose your favorite fruits, like berries, mangoes, or peaches. Puree the fruits in a blender until smooth and combine them with plain, unsweetened Greek yogurt. You can use a small amount of honey or maple syrup to add some sweetness without making migraines worse. Spoon the mixture into silicone molds or ice cube trays and freeze until solid.

These layered bites look good and taste good too! The combination of creamy yogurt and sweet fruit makes for a satisfying and refreshing treat. To create a layered effect, alternate layers of yogurt and fruit puree. To begin, add a spoonful of pureed fruit into each mold, then top it with a layer of yogurt. Continue layering until the molds are full. Freeze the trays for several hours or overnight.

These bites become mini frozen yogurt popsicles that are easy to handle and eat, which makes them even more kid-friendly and fun! These treats are great for hot days or as a healthy snack any time of year, and they provide a balanced combination of protein from the yogurt and vitamins from the fruit, making them a nutritious option for migraine sufferers. You can also insert small popsicle sticks into each mold before freezing.

A great option for a quick and simple treat that won't heat your kitchen is no-bake dessert bars. To make the base, combine crushed nuts, oats, and a natural sweetener such as honey or maple syrup. Mix these ingredients with a small amount of melted coconut oil until they form a cohesive mixture. Press this mixture firmly into the bottom of a lined baking dish to form the crust. You can also add some shredded coconut or cocoa powder for extra flavor and texture.

These bars can have a variety of migraine-friendly fillings, but a popular one is a peanut butter and honey filling, which is made by blending natural peanut butter, honey, and a small amount of vanilla extract until it's smooth and spreads evenly over the crust.

If you want to add a layer of chocolate, melt some dark chocolate and pour it over the peanut butter layer, using a spatula to spread it evenly. Refrigerate the bars for a few hours until they solidify.

For a fruity twist, puree your favorite fruit (strawberries, blueberries, etc.) and stir into Greek yogurt to make a sticky, dough-like consistency. Press this mixture into the bottom of your dish. Spread the fruity yogurt mixture over the date and almond base. Chill the bars in the fridge until they are set. Slice into squares and serve for a cool, healthful no-bake dessert.

REVIVING FRUIT POPS AND SORBET

Since they don't contain dairy or artificial additives, sorbet and fruit pops are refreshing and light desserts that are ideal for people who suffer from migraines. To make a basic fruit sorbet, first, puree some fresh or frozen fruit in a blender until it's smooth.

If necessary, add a little honey or agave syrup to taste it even more. Then, pour the puree into an ice cream maker and churn it according to the manufacturer's instructions. If you don't have an ice cream maker, you can pour the mixture into a shallow dish and freeze it, stirring it every 30 minutes until it becomes sorbet-like.

Fruit pops are a great treat for controlling hydration levels, which is important for preventing migraines. To make fruit pops, blend fresh fruits like watermelon, strawberries, or pineapple until smooth. Pour the puree into popsicle molds and insert sticks. You can add small chunks of fruit into the molds before pouring in the puree for a more interesting texture. Freeze the molds for several hours or overnight until solid.

Layered fruit pops are easily made and customized so that you always have a healthy, migraine-friendly dessert option on hand. Simply fill the molds halfway with one fruit puree, freeze until slightly firm, then add another fruit puree on top and freeze again. This results in gorgeous, multi-layered pops that are visually appealing and enjoyable to eat. You can experiment with different combinations like mango and raspberry or kiwi and blueberry.

BAKED FRUIT COBBLERS AND CRISPS

The right ingredients can make baked fruit crisps and cobblers migraine-friendly. To start, choose fruits that are less likely to cause migraines, like apples, pears, or blueberries. Peel and slice the fruits, then toss them with a little lemon juice, honey, and cinnamon. Evenly spread the fruit mixture in a baking dish.

This dessert is best served warm and goes well with a scoop of vanilla Greek yogurt for extra creaminess. To make the crisp topping, combine rolled oats, almond flour, and a small amount of brown sugar or a natural sweetener. Add a little melted coconut oil or butter and stir until the mixture becomes crumbly. Spread the topping evenly over the fruit. Bake in a preheated oven at 350°F (175°C) for about 30 minutes, or until the topping is golden brown and the fruit is bubbling.

A different topping is used for cobblers, which are made with almond flour, baking powder, and salt. In another bowl, beat together an egg, melted butter, and a small amount of honey or maple syrup to create a thick batter. Drop spoonfuls of the batter over the fruit filling, spreading it out evenly.

RECIPES FOR HYDRATING INFUSED WATER

To maximize the release of flavors and nutrients from fresh fruits, vegetables, and herbs like cucumber, lemon, mint, berries, and ginger, thinly slice and wash them. Then, combine your chosen ingredients in a large pitcher of cold water and refrigerate for at least two hours to allow the flavors to fully infuse. Making hydrating-infused water recipes is an easy yet effective way to ensure adequate hydration while enjoying various flavors and potential health benefits.

Try blending different combinations until you find your favorite: cucumber, mint, and lemon make a refreshing and purifying drink; berries and basil make a sweet and aromatic drink; you can even add a small pinch of salt for electrolyte balance, which is especially helpful in hot weather or after working out. Drink the infused water within 24 to 48 hours to maintain freshness and stop bacteria from growing.

Serve the infused water in clear glasses with a few of the fruit and herb slices inside for a more visually appealing presentation. This will not only make the drink more appealing but will also encourage regular hydration. Infused waters are a great substitute for sugary drinks and can help relieve dehydration, which is a common migraine trigger. You can support overall health and well-being by regularly drinking these flavorful and hydrating waters.

HERBAL TEA COMBINATIONS TO ALLEVIATE MIGRAINES

Because they naturally contain anti-inflammatory and calming properties, herbal teas can be a calming and effective way to manage migraines. To make your herbal tea blends start with premium dried herbs like feverfew, chamomile, peppermint, and ginger, which are well-known for their ability to relieve migraines. Measure out one to two teaspoons of each herb for each cup of tea you wish to brew, adjusting the ratios based on your taste preferences and the specific effects you seek.

In a teapot or infuser, combine the dried herbs with boiling water; let steep for 5 to 10 minutes, allowing the herbs to release their health benefits; strain tea into a cup and enjoy warm; you can add a little honey or a slice of lemon to enhance the flavor.

Regular use of herbal tea blends can help reduce migraine frequency and severity by inducing relaxation and reducing inflammation.

Herbal teas are a gentle yet effective tool in your migraine management toolkit. For convenience, make larger batches of your favorite blends and store them in airtight containers so you can quickly brew a cup whenever you feel a migraine coming on.

You can also experiment with different herb combinations to find what works best for you. For example, a blend of chamomile and lavender can be particularly calming, while ginger and peppermint can provide a more invigorating effect.

A base of leafy greens, like spinach or kale, which are rich in magnesium, a mineral known to help reduce migraine frequency, is a great way to make sure you are getting a variety of vitamins and minerals that can help prevent migraines. Add a serving of fruit, like bananas, berries, or mangoes, to provide natural sweetness and a good dose of antioxidants.

To enhance the nutritional value of this smoothie, add some healthy fats and proteins (like avocado, Greek yogurt, or a scoop of protein powder) to help keep you full and stabilize blood sugar, which can be a migraine trigger. You can also add some omega-3 fatty acids (like chia, flax, or hemp) to the smoothie by adding a handful of these nuts or seeds, which can further support brain health. Finally, blend everything with a cup of your favorite liquid (like almond milk, coconut water, or plain water) until everything is well combined.

Consistency is key when it comes to ensuring that the macronutrient balance and variety of ingredients cover different nutritional bases. Regular consumption of these nutrient-dense smoothies can help maintain overall health and possibly reduce the incidence of migraines. Enjoy these smoothies as part of your daily routine, especially as a breakfast option or a mid-day snack.

ENERGIZING TYPES OF TEA AND COFFEE

Choosing high-quality coffee beans or tea leaves can maximize the benefits of energizing coffee and tea varieties. For coffee, consider methods like French press or pour-over, which allow better control over the brewing process and can result in a richer, more flavorful cup. Caffeine in moderation can help relieve migraine symptoms for some people by constricting blood vessels and reducing inflammation.

Try teas that are high in antioxidants and caffeine, like black tea, green tea, or matcha. Green tea is a great option because it gives you a subtle energy boost without the jitters that come with higher caffeine levels.

Matcha is a powdered form of green tea that is particularly strong and can be whisked into hot water or milk for a creamy, energizing drink.

If you are sensitive to caffeine, you may want to consider decaffeinated coffee or herbal teas like rooibos, which offer a similar experience without the stimulant effects. By selecting the right coffee and tea varieties and consuming them in moderation, you can enjoy their energizing benefits while managing your migraine triggers effectively. You should also minimize overindulgence in these beverages to avoid sleep disturbances, which can be another cause of migraines.

FRESHLY PREPARED COCKTAILS AND JUICES

Make a base of fresh, seasonal fruits and vegetables (carrots, beets, apples, and leafy greens like spinach or kale are excellent choices because of their high vitamin and mineral content) and use a juicer to extract the pure juice from these ingredients, ensuring you get the maximum nutrients in an easily digestible form. Freshly made mocktails and juices are refreshing and can provide essential nutrients that support overall health and migraine prevention.

Mocktails can be made by blending these freshly squeezed juices with sparkling water or coconut water for a little extra hydration and fizz. You can also play around with flavorings and add extra therapeutic benefits, such as a refreshing blend of beet juice, apple juice, and a dash of ginger that also supports cardiovascular health, which is important for managing migraines.

These juices and mocktails make a healthy substitute for sugary sodas and alcoholic beverages, which can trigger migraines. By adding a variety of fruits, vegetables, and herbs to your juice and mocktail recipes, you can enjoy delicious, hydrating beverages that support your health and help prevent migraines. Serve these drinks chilled, with ice, and garnished with fresh fruit slices or herbs for a visually appealing presentation.

CHAPTER FOUR

MENUS FOR SPECIAL OCCASIONS

RECIPES FOR HOLIDAYS AND CELEBRATIONS

It can be fun and fulfilling to prepare migraine-friendly meals for special occasions like holidays. To begin, concentrate on using whole, fresh ingredients to make tasty dishes free of common migraine triggers. Choose lean proteins like chicken or turkey, and use fresh herbs and spices rather than pre-packaged seasoning mixes to make sure there are no hidden additives. Roasted vegetables, quinoa salads, and mashed sweet potatoes are good choices for side dishes because they are healthy and unlikely to cause migraines.

Desserts are a little trickier, but still doable: homemade fruit desserts, like baked apples with cinnamon or a berry compote, can be festive and migraine-friendly since they don't include chocolate, aged cheeses, or artificial sweeteners—all of which are common migraine triggers.

You can also bake your own baked goods with migraine-friendly flour and natural sweeteners like honey or maple syrup to enjoy sweet treats without guilt.

Careful planning and selection of ingredients can help you enjoy holiday and celebration meals without jeopardizing your health. Beverages: Steer clear of alcohol and caffeine, as these are common triggers for many migraine sufferers. Instead, offer herbal teas, infused water with fresh fruit, or homemade lemonade. These drinks can be refreshing and add a festive touch without raising the risk of a migraine attack.

STYLISH MENUS FOR DINNER PARTIES

A migraine diet requires careful planning and inventive recipe development to create an elegant dinner party that will wow your guests and keep you safe from triggers. Start with a sophisticated appetizer like roasted red pepper hummus or chilled cucumber soup served with fresh vegetables; these dishes are flavorful, light, and free of common migraine triggers like aged cheeses and processed meats.

Choose a main course that consists of grilled fish or chicken with a fresh herb marinade, served with quinoa pilaf and a side of roasted seasonal vegetables. Safe options for fish include salmon or tilapia, which can be flavored with herbs like basil, thyme, and rosemary. Roasted vegetables can include bell peppers, carrots, and asparagus. Quinoa is a hearty and migraine-friendly base.

With these thoughtful selections, you can host an elegant dinner party that everyone will enjoy, even those who manage migraines. For dessert, think of something elegant but still simple, like a poached pear with a drizzle of honey or a fresh fruit salad with a hint of mint.

These options are both visually appealing and satisfying, and they avoid common dessert ingredients that can trigger migraines. To round out the meal, serve non-alcoholic sparkling water with a splash of natural fruit juice or herbal teas to keep the beverage selection safe and pleasant.

SEASONAL OFFERS FOR DIETS TREATING MIGRAINES

Using seasonal ingredients in your diet can make your meals more interesting and varied. In the spring and summer, try lighter, fresh recipes like chilled gazpacho made from ripe tomatoes, cucumbers, and bell peppers or a strawberry and spinach salad dressed with a lemon vinaigrette; these recipes bring out the flavors of the season without resorting to common migraine triggers like aged cheeses and processed dressings.

Heartier fare, like quinoa and roasted vegetable bake or roasted butternut squash soup with a hint of nutmeg, can be featured on fall and winter menus. These dishes take advantage of the seasonal produce and are warm and comforting without making you feel like you're suffering from a migraine. For a festive touch, try a spiced apple cider, which can be served hot or cold and made with fresh apples, cinnamon, and cloves.

Desserts are seasonal and can be just as delicious. For example, in the summer, try a refreshing watermelon sorbet made from pureed watermelon and a little honey; in the winter, bake an apple with a dollop of plain yogurt and a sprinkle of cinnamon for a safe and comforting treat. By planning your menu accordingly, you can have a delicious and varied migraine-friendly diet all year long.

BIRTHDAY AND ANNIVERSARY SWEETS

A homemade vanilla cake with fresh fruit topping can be both festive and safe, avoiding chocolate and artificial flavors which can be triggers. Celebrating birthdays and anniversaries on a migraine diet doesn't mean you have to miss out on delicious treats. For cakes and pastries, consider using alternative flours like almond or coconut flour, and natural sweeteners like honey or maple syrup.

Consider creating individual desserts such as fruit parfaits or mini tarts for more individualized treats.

A visually striking and delicious dessert can be made by layering fresh berries with a dollop of whipped coconut cream. Mini tarts made with a gluten-free crust and filled with a creamy, dairy-free filling and topped with fresh fruit can also be a hit, providing both flavor and migraine safety.

Another way to celebrate without running the risk of a migraine is to provide small bites or snacks, such as almonds, fresh fruit slices, and homemade energy bars made with oats, seeds, and dried fruit. These are not only healthy, but they also help avoid common migraine triggers, such as artificial additives and processed snacks. With a little imagination, you can make sure that birthdays and anniversaries are marked with happiness and delectable, migraine-safe treats.

ADVICE FOR SAFE DINING OUT

Managing a migraine diet while dining out can be difficult, but it can be done safely with careful planning and communication. Look for restaurants that specialize in fresh, whole foods and have a good reputation for working with dietary restrictions; many now offer their menus online so you can see what's safe to eat before you get there.

Speak with the server or chef when you arrive at the restaurant about your dietary requirements and explain that you must stay away from certain trigger foods, such as aged cheeses, processed meats, and artificial additives. Don't be afraid to inquire about ingredient lists and preparation techniques. To reduce the possibility of hidden triggers, choose simple dishes like grilled meats or fish, steamed vegetables, and salads dressed with olive oil and vinegar.

Being proactive and prepared will allow you to enjoy dining out without worrying about inciting a migraine attack. Finally, always have a backup plan. Carry safe snacks like nuts or a piece of fruit in case you can't find suitable options on the menu. Additionally, drink plenty of water to stay hydrated and avoid beverages that can trigger migraines, like alcohol and caffeinated drinks.

CHAPTER FIVE

CONTROLLING STRESS AND SLEEP TO PREVENT MIGRAINES

Stress is a common trigger for migraines, so it's important to incorporate relaxation techniques into your daily routine. Activities like yoga, deep breathing exercises, and mindfulness meditation can significantly reduce stress levels. Making time each day for these activities can help you manage the stressors that could potentially trigger a migraine and create a sense of calm.

Another important component of preventing migraines is practicing good sleep hygiene. Be consistent in going to bed and waking up at the same times every day, including on the weekends. Establish a soothing bedtime routine that tells your body when it's time to unwind. Avoid screens and stimulants like caffeine close to bedtime. Make sure your sleeping environment is cool, dark, and quiet.

These actions help your body's internal clock to be more in tune with itself, which improves the quality of your sleep and lowers your risk of migraines.

Managing your stress and maintaining proper sleep hygiene can work in concert to prevent migraines. Other supportive factors in this strategy include regular exercise, eating a balanced diet, and drinking plenty of water. When you put these things first, you establish a whole-home environment that reduces stress and promotes restorative sleep, which in turn reduces the frequency and intensity of migraine attacks.

THE BENEFITS OF EXERCISE FOR LOWERING FREQUENCY OF MIGRAINES

Exercise helps regulate many bodily systems, including the release of endorphins, which are natural painkillers and mood elevators. Aerobic exercises, such as walking, cycling, and swimming, are particularly effective in this regard. Aim for at least 30 minutes of moderate exercise most days of the week to reap the full benefits.

Regular physical activity is a powerful tool in reducing the frequency and severity of migraines.

When adding exercise to your migraine management plan, consistency is key. If you're not used to regular physical activity, start slowly and gradually increase the intensity and duration. To keep yourself motivated, choose activities you enjoy. You can also prevent exercise-induced migraines by staying hydrated and warming up properly before exercise. Finally, making sure your physical activity is both enjoyable and beneficial requires careful planning.

Exercise has many physical advantages, but it also helps reduce stress, which is a major migraine trigger. Physical activity regularly can enhance sleep quality, which is another important migraine prevention factor. By incorporating regular exercise into your routine, you not only enhance your general health but also build a strong defense against migraine onset.

For people who experience migraines, it's critical to recognize and control triggers. Common triggers include aged cheeses, alcohol, and processed meats, which contain chemicals like tyramine and nitrates. You can identify specific triggers by keeping a food diary, which will help you modify your diet to avoid these migraine inducers.

Understanding your sensitivities can help you take proactive steps to minimize exposure. For example, wearing sunglasses in bright sunlight, avoiding strong perfumes, and creating a quiet, calming environment can reduce the likelihood of a migraine attack. Environmental factors also play a significant role in triggering migraines. Weather changes, bright lights, strong smells, and loud noises can all contribute to the onset of a migraine.

Other common triggers include stress and hormonal changes, which can be effectively managed with stress management techniques and a consistent sleep schedule. For women, hormonal fluctuations associated with the menstrual cycle can be particularly significant, so tracking your cycle and talking with a healthcare provider about preventative strategies can help manage these hormonal triggers.

One commonly asked question is about the role of caffeine in migraines. While small amounts of caffeine can occasionally relieve migraine symptoms, excessive consumption or withdrawal can trigger migraines. To effectively manage the effects of caffeine, it's important to monitor your intake and understand how your body responds to it. A migraine diet focuses on identifying and avoiding foods that may trigger attacks.

Another common question is what kinds of foods are best for a migraine diet. Generally speaking, fresh, whole foods like a range of fruits, vegetables, lean proteins, and whole grains are advised because they contain vital nutrients and antioxidants that can help reduce inflammation and prevent migraines. It's also important to stay hydrated throughout the day because dehydration is known to trigger migraines.

A lot of people are curious about certain dietary approaches, like the ketogenic diet or elimination diets. Although some people find relief with these diets, it's best to speak with a healthcare professional or nutritionist before making major dietary changes. They can help you navigate the process and make sure you continue to eat a healthy, balanced diet while recognizing and avoiding potential migraine triggers.

SOURCES & ADDITIONAL READING

Books such as Tara Spencer's "The Migraine Relief Diet" and David Buchholz's "Heal Your Headache" offer thorough guides on identifying triggers and managing symptoms through dietary adjustments. These resources not only provide practical tips and recipes tailored to migraine sufferers but can also be very helpful for those looking for more information on managing migraines through diet and lifestyle changes.

Websites like the American Migraine Foundation and Migraine.com provide a wealth of information, including articles, research updates, and community forums where people can exchange experiences and recommendations. These sites help learn about the most recent advancements in migraine research and connect with other people who have experienced the condition.

Speaking with medical specialists, such as neurologists and dietitians, can also be helpful. They can offer tailored recommendations and treatment programs based on your circumstances and past medical records. Using these services guarantees a comprehensive migraine management strategy that combines professional advice with doable, everyday tactics for avoidance and alleviation.

www.ingramcontent.com/pod-product-compliance
Lightning Source LLC
Chambersburg PA
CBHW061251250726
48653CB00002B/604